Midwifery Client File

Client Name:

EDD:

ACCOUNT LEDGER

Name: _____ Phone: _____

Address: _____

Initial service date: _____ EDD: _____

Agreements

Agreed Fee: _____ Non-Refundable Deposit: _____ Assistant Fee: _____

Services to include: _____

Payment Plan: _____

Miscellaneous

Assistant Fee and Date Paid: _____

Other Fee and Date Paid: _____

DATE	DESCRIPTION	CASH	CHECK #	AMOUNT	BALANCE DUE

Registration Form

_____   _____   _____
Name of Client (First/Middle/Last)   (Maiden)   Date of Birth

_____   _____
Father's Name (First/Middle/Last)   Father's Date of Birth

_____   _____
Client's Occupation   Father's Occupation

_____
Complete Address

_____
Mailing Address (if different)

(_____)_____   (_____)_____   (_____)_____
Home Phone   Cellular Phone   Other (specify):

_____
E-mail Address

_____   _____
Insurance Carrier   Policy Number and Date of Effectiveness

Are you the primary insured? _____ If not who is? _____ Relationship_____

_____
Insurance Address

(_____)_____
Insurance Phone

In case of an emergency, is there anyone you would want us to contact? Please list their contact information/phone numbers:

_____

_____

_____

_____

_____

Personal GYN History for _____

Menstrual History

How often do you menstruate? _____days
Is your flow ☐ scant ☐ moderate ☐ heavy ☐ regular ☐ irreg
If irregular, please explain
_____

How old were you when you started menstruating?_____
Do you have cramps? YES NO ☐ mild ☐ moderate ☐ severe
When was your last menstrual period?_____
Was it normal?_____
Are you aware of the date you conceived?_____

Gynecological & Birth Control History

When was your last pap smear?_____
Have you ever had an abnormal pap smear? YES NO_____

Have you ever had   infertility_____   vag inf_____
  abnormal bleeding_____   breast surgery_____
  cervical surgery_____   uterine surgery_____
  Any STDs_____
Do you feel that you might be at risk for any STDs? YES NO

Most recent birth control used_____
Contraception used in the past; what, when, any problems?
_____
_____
_____

Sexual History

Are you sexually active YES NO
Do you have painful intercourse? YES NO Bleeding? YES NO
How would you describe your sexual relationship?_____
_____
How do you feel your sexual relationship has changed since
you got pregnant?_____
_____
Have you had more than one partner? YES NO
Have you ever had non consensual sex? YES NO
If so, do you feel that experience will affect have an affect on
your labor/birth?_____

Was this a planned pregnancy? YES NO
What are your feelings about it?_____
Your spouse's/partner's feelings?_____

Anything else?

Anything else you would like me to know?

Client's Pregnancy History (list all pregnancies and outcomes)

DOB	Name	M/F	How many weeks	Weight	Hours Labor	c-sec/ vbac	Any issues or complications during pregnancy or birth?

Problems in Current Pregnancy

☐ 1st trimester nausea_____
☐ 2nd/3rd trimester nausea_____
☐ Varicose veins_____
☐ Bladder infections_____
☐ Kidney infections_____
☐ Spotting/Bleeding_____
☐ Premature labor_____
☐ Anemia_____

☐ Constipation_____
☐ Hemorrhoids_____
☐ Headaches_____
☐ Dizziness_____
☐ Swelling_____
☐ Gastritis_____
☐ Heartburn_____
☐ Any trauma_____

Exposures in Current Pregnancy

☐ Tobacco_____
☐ Alcohol_____
☐ Caffeine_____
☐ Marijuana_____
☐ Cocaine_____
☐ Street Drugs_____
☐ Other meds_____
☐ Non-pres.drugs_____

☐ Vitamins_____
☐ Fumes/sprays_____
☐ Enviro Toxins_____
☐ X-rays_____
☐ Measles/Viruses_____
☐ Vaccinations_____
☐ Cats_____
☐ Other_____

_____

Social History

Do you enjoy your work? YES NO _____
Describe your stress level_____
_____

What do you do to relax or relieve stress?_____
Do you exercise? YES NO How often?_____ How long?____
Tobacco Use ☐ None Packs/Day_____ How long?_____
Do you want to quit smoking? YES NO
Street Drug Use ☐ None Drug_____ How often?_____
Alcohol Use ☐ None # Drinks/Day/Week/Month_____

Have you ever been or are you now in an abusive
relationship? YES NO

Has anyone now, or in the past :
Hit, kicked or pushed you? YES NO
Verbally abused you? YES NO

Do you feel safe in your current relationship? YES NO

EMOTIONAL RISK ASSESSMENT

Are you a nervous person? YES NO
Do you often feel sad or depressed? YES NO
Do you feel a desire to hurt others? YES NO

Do you often feel angry or upset? YES NO
Do you feel a desire to hurt yourself? YES NO
Have you recently suffered a major loss/change? YES NO
Is there anything else you feel could be helpful to us in
providing your care? _____

Client's Medical History

Allergies to any medications?_____ Reactions_____
Have you ever had a blood transfusion? YES NO   Any uterine surgeries? _____
List any other injuries, surgery, or hospitalization with dates_____

Check all that apply:

☐ Asthma_____	☐ Seizures_____	☐ Auto immune disorders____	☐ Liver problems_____
☐ Diabetes_____	☐ Thrombophlebitis_____	☐ Cancer_____	☐ Blood disorders_____
☐ Drug addiction_____	☐ Chronic Hypertension_____	☐ TB_____	☐ HIV / Hepatitis_____
☐ Heart disease_____	☐ Renal disease_____	☐ Thyroid disorder_____	☐ Syphilis_____

Risk Assessment

In this or one of your previous pregnancies have you had:

YES NO Severe hyperemesis requiring hospitalization
YES NO Preterm rupture of membranes (<36 wks)
YES NO Shoulder dystocia, resulting in trauma to the baby
YES NO Placenta abruption
YES NO Placenta previa
YES NO Gestational diabetes (controlled)
YES NO RH sensitization
YES NO Medical disorders or endocrine, renal, cardiac or
        vascular systems

YES NO Postpartum hemorrhage (requiring bl transfusion)
YES NO Pelvic/genital tract abnormalities
YES NO Suspected cervical incompetence
YES NO Inverted uterus
YES NO Recurrent UTI's

YES NO Are you or the FOB related by blood?
YES NO Are your or the FOB from any of these ethnic/racial
        groups? Jewish Black/African Asian Mediterranean

Family's Medical History

Father: Alive and well? YES NO_____ Mother: Alive and well? YES NO_____ Siblings: Alive and well? YES NO_____

Check all that apply:

☐ Hypertension_____	☐ Heart disease_____	☐ Allergies_____	☐ Downs syndrome_____
☐ Kidney problems_____	☐ Blood disorders_____	☐ Twins_____	☐ Cancer_____
☐ Diabetes_____	☐ TB_____	☐ Genetic anomalies_____	☐ Other_____

Client Health Record Checklist

Name _____   EDD _____

INITIAL VISIT

_____ Draw Labs
_____ AFP ☐ Declined ☐ To do
_____ CF ☐ Declined ☐ To do
_____ Genetic Counseling, PRN
_____ Diet History
_____ Danger Signs
_____ Habits: smoking, ETOH, drugs
_____ Exercise; sexuality
_____ Discomforts
_____ Financial Agreement
_____ Consent Forms

16-20 WEEKS

_____ Schedule US, PRN
_____ Draw/Decline AFP

24-28 WEEKS

_____ Draw/Decline GT
_____ HCT
_____ AB screen PRN
_____ Rhogam PRN
_____ PTL Signs
_____ Childbirth Class
_____ Breastfeeding

30-32 WEEKS

_____ Labor Support
_____ Danger Signs: ROM, headache, visual disturbances, etc

34-36 WEEKS

_____ Obtain/Decline Group B Strep
_____ Supplies & preparation list

36 WEEKS

_____ Signs of Labor
_____ When and How to Call
_____ Pediatrician
_____ Supplies
_____ PP Support
_____ Breastfeeding
_____ Ready for Baby
_____ Back-up Plan/Map
_____ Newborn Screen Information

Continues to Meet Risk Criteria for Birth Home
(Weekly Evaluation)

36	37	38	39	40	41	42
☐	☐	☐	☐	☐	☐	☐

40-42 WEEKS

_____ Post-dates Routine
_____ NST
_____ Kick Count

RECORDS

Records Requested: _____
Records Received: _____

Lab Tests and Results

Client ID

Client Name

Date and Time	Tests Ordered	Results Received Date	Results

Lab Tests and Results

Client ID

Client Name

Date and Time	Tests Ordered	Results Received Date	Results

Ultrasound Exams and Reults

Client ID

Client Name

Date and Time	Tests Ordered	Results Received Date	Results

Client Name	Age		Meds		Allergies/Reaction	
	Height					
Date of Birth	Weight					
	LMP					
P SAB TAB L	BP					
Reason for Visit	Hgb				Food:	
	Tobacco Y N					

Interval History

Physical Exam   Date   Initials

Gen Health	Physical			Height		Weight	BMI
	Emotional/Abuse/DV			Blood Pressure		Pulse	Temp

HEENT	Head ❏WNL	Lymph Glands ❏WNL		Eyes	Sclera ❏WNL
	Neck ❏WNL	Ears ❏WNL			Conjunctiva ❏WNL
	Thyroid ❏WNL	Nose/Mouth ❏WNL			Pupil Reaction ❏WNL

Chest

Breast Exam ❏Performed ❏Taught ❏Monthly BSE Advised ❏Discussed Mammograms ❏Nipples Checked
Comments:

Heart	Rate	Rhythm	Sounds	Lungs	Respiration Rate	Sounds

Abdomen & Back	Bowel Sounds	Spleen	Liver	Masses	Diastasis FB	Scars
	Inguinal Nodes	Femoral Pulses	CVAT		Kidneys	Spine
	Fundal Height CM	Placental Sounds (o)	Fetal Motion	FHT BPM	Fetal Position	Location of FHT

Extre-mities	Edema	Lesions	Reflexes	Clonus	Varicose Veins	Joint Range of Motion	Bruises

Skin	Tone	Lesions	Lumps	Color	Rash	Hair	Nails

Genitourinary	External		Internal	
	Scars ❏Y ❏N		Uterus ❏Anteflexed ❏Retroflexed	
	Prolapse ❏Y ❏N		❏ Normal Size, Shape, Contour	
	Discharge ❏Y ❏N		Cervix ❏WNL ❏ PAP Performed	
	Erythema ❏Y ❏N		Ovaries Palpable ❏Y ❏N ❏Possible Cyst	
	Sx of STDs/Infection ❏Y ❏N		Vagina ❏Cystocele ❏Rectocele ❏WNL	
	Anus/Rectum ❏WNL Lesions/Scars/Fissures/Hemorrhoids/Inflammation			
	Comments			

Assessment

Plan

Midwife   **Assistants**

Prenatal Record

Mother _____

Partner _____

Children _____

Special Concerns & Considerations

_____

_____

_____

G	P	T	P	Sa	Ea	L

LMP _____

EDD: (N/W/US) _____

DOB _____

Blood Type _____

Allergies _____

Pre-pregnancy Weight _____

DATE	WEEKS	WEIGHT	BP/PULSE	FUNDUS	POSITION	FHT	MOVE MENT	URINE Pr/Gl/WBC		RETURN VISIT	INITIALS
									BA Bleeding Discharge Dizzy Edema Elimination Fatigue Gastric HA Mood N&V Sleep Vision Varicosities UC Urine		
									BA Bleeding Discharge Dizzy Edema Elimination Fatigue Gastric HA Mood N&V Sleep Vision Varicosities UC Urine		
									BA Bleeding Discharge Dizzy Edema Elimination Fatigue Gastric HA Mood N&V Sleep Vision Varicosities UC Urine		
									BA Bleeding Discharge Dizzy Edema Elimination Fatigue Gastric HA Mood N&V Sleep Vision Varicosities UC Urine		
									BA Bleeding Discharge Dizzy Edema Elimination Fatigue Gastric HA Mood N&V Sleep Vision Varicosities UC Urine		
									BA Bleeding Discharge Dizzy Edema Elimination Fatigue Gastric HA Mood N&V Sleep Vision Varicosities UC Urine		
									BA Bleeding Discharge Dizzy Edema Elimination Fatigue Gastric HA Mood N&V Sleep Vision Varicosities UC Urine		
									BA Bleeding Discharge Dizzy Edema Elimination Fatigue Gastric HA Mood N&V Sleep Vision Varicosities UC Urine		
									BA Bleeding Discharge Dizzy Edema Elimination Fatigue Gastric HA Mood N&V Sleep Vision Varicosities UC Urine		
									BA Bleeding Discharge Dizzy Edema Elimination Fatigue Gastric HA Mood N&V Sleep Vision Varicosities UC Urine		
									BA Bleeding Discharge Dizzy Edema Elimination Fatigue Gastric HA Mood N&V Sleep Vision Varicosities UC Urine		
									BA Bleeding Discharge Dizzy Edema Elimination Fatigue Gastric HA Mood N&V Sleep Vision Varicosities UC Urine		
									BA Bleeding Discharge Dizzy Edema Elimination Fatigue Gastric HA Mood N&V Sleep Vision Varicosities UC Urine		

Prenatal Follow Up Sheet for _____

G_____ P_____ A_____ L_____ EDD_____ Revised_____

Date	Issues Discussed	Midwife	Student

Prenatal Follow Up Sheet for _____

G_____ P_____ A_____ L_____ EDD_____ Revised_____

Date	Issues Discussed	Midwife	Student

Prenatal Follow Up Sheet for _____

G_____ P_____ A_____ L_____ EDD_____ Revised_____

Date	Issues Discussed	Midwife	Student

Labor Initial Intake

Client Name:_____ **Phone#**:_____

Significant Issues:_____

Age:_____ **Gest. Wks**:_____ G/P:_____ EDD:_____ **Blood Type**:_____

SROM:_____ **Time**:_____ **Colour**:_____ **Odour**:_____ Show:_____

Time CTX Began:_____ Spacing:_____ Lasting:_____ Coping:_____

Eating:_____ Drinking:_____ Time Last Eaten:_____ Voiding:_____ BM:_____

TEMP	PULSE	BP	FHT	FUNDUS	POSITION	OTHER
					Movement	

Client's Concerns:_____
_____
_____

Notes

Midwife Staying?:_____ Transport to Hosp.?:_____
Early Labour Handout Given:_____ Has Labour/Birth Supplies:_____
Support People:_____

Prenatal Issues		
BP Range:	**BP Limits:**	**Any s/s PIH?**
Consults:	Completed:	Outstanding:
Hemo:	Varicosities:	**Labs WNL:**
FHR Range:	Fetal Probs:	Other:
Emotional:	Nutr./Vits.:	Hx of SA/Mol:
# Appts:	Complied Recos:	All Waivers Signed:

Client Name					Partner				Midwife		
Allergies						Blood Type	GBS Status + - ?		Assistant(s)		
G	P	SAB	TAB	L	VBAC Y N		LMP			EDD	

Onset of Labor	Date/Time	Contractions	Membranes	Show	Fetal Movement	Time MW Called	Comments

Assessment at Arrival	Date/Time	Contractions	Membranes	Show	Fetal Movement	Comments
	B/P	Pulse	Temp	Internal Exam	Activity/Rest/Food/Drink	

Time	B/P	Pulse	Temp	FHT Rate Variability Location	IN	Out	Contractions Frequency (Minutes)	Duration (Seconds)	Internal Exam Dilation Station Effacement Position	Comments	Initials

Client Name	Date	Midwife/Students

Time	B/P	Pulse	Temp	FHT	IN	Out	Contractions		Internal Exam	Comments	Initials
				Rate Variability Location			Frequency (Minutes)	Duration (Seconds)	**Dilation** **Station** **Effacement** **Position**		

Client Name					Date				Midwife/Students		

Time	B/P	Pulse	Temp	FHT	IN	Out	Contractions		Internal Exam	Comments	Initials
				Rate Variability Location			Frequency (Minutes)	Duration (Seconds)	Dilation Station Effacement Position		

Labor Notes for _____

Baby's Name_____ Date of Birth_____

Date	Issues Discussed	Midwife	Student

Labor Notes for _____

Baby's Name _____ Date of Birth _____

Date	Issues Discussed	Midwife	Student

Labor Notes for _____

Baby's Name_____ Date of Birth_____

Date	Issues Discussed	Midwife	Student

Immediate Postpartum Record

Date:_____ Time of birth:_____ am/pm

Client's Status (name)_____

Time	Vitals			Uterus PBL_____cups/cc		In/Out	Comments	Init
Hour am/pm	Pulse	Temp	B/P	Status	Blood loss	Intake, etc	Notes	Initials

Baby's Status (name)_____

Time	Vitals			In/Out		Comments	Init
Hour am/pm	Pulse	Resp	Temp	Intake	Output	Notes	Initials

Total time of postpartum care_____ Total estimated blood loss_____

Discharged from Midwife's care on_____ at _____ am/pm MW_____

Newborn Exam

Baby's Name			Mother's Name			
Date		Time	APGAR	1 Minute	5 Minutes	Sign
Gender	Weight	Length	Heart Rate			0 = Absent 1 = Below 100 2 = Above 100
OFC	Chest	EGA	Respiratory Effort			0 = Absent 1 = Slow, Irregular 2 = Good crying
Respirations	Heart Rate	Temp	Muscle Tone			0 = Flaccid 1 = Some flexion of extremities 2 = Active motion
Birth Time	Midwife		Color			0 = Pale blue 1 = Body pink, extremities blue 2 = Completely pink
General Appearance (activity, tone, cry)			Reflex Irritability			0 = None 1 = Grimace 2 = Vigorous Cry
			Total Score			

Skin (polycythemia, jaundice desquamation, lanugo, birth marks)

Head. Neck (molding, caput, bruising, cephalhematoma, fontanelles)

Eyes (red spots, jaundice, pupils, tracking)	Erythromycin Ointment
ENT (ear placement, reactivity to sound, lips, palate, frenulum)	Hips (clicks, creases)
Thorax (retractions) Present? Y / N	Abdomen (cord, masses)
Heart	Femoral Pulses
Genitals (testes descended, edema, labia, clitoris)	Spine/Anus (sinuses, anus patent)
Lungs	Extremities (fingers, toes, clavicles)

Reflexes

Babinski	Present?	Y / N	Sucking	Present?	Y / N	Comments
Palmar	Present?	Y / N	Swallowing	Present?	Y / N	
Plantar	Present?	Y / N	Step	Present?	Y / N	
Moro	Present?	Y / N	Tonic Neck	Present?	Y / N	

Gestational Age Assessment (in weeks)	Preterm				Term				Post-term	
	34	35	36	37	38	39	40	41	42	43+
Vernix	Covers body, thick layer				Back, scalp, in creases		Scant in creases		No vernix	
Breast Tissue and Areola	Areola raised		1-2 mm nodule		3-5 mm	5-6 mm	7-10 mm			
Ear Form	Beginning incurving superior		Incurving upper 2/3 pinnae		Well-defined incurving to lobe					
Ear Cartilage	Scant, ret. slowly from folding		Thin, springs back from folding				Pinnae firm, remains erect from head			
Sole Creases	1-2 ant.	2-3 ant.	Anterior 2/3 sole		Involving heel				Entire sole	
Skin (thickness and appearance)	Smooth, no edema		Thicker, no desquamation, few vessels				Some desquamation		Thick, desq entire body	
Nail plates	Nails to fingertips								Well past tips	
Hair	Fine/wooly, bunches out from head				Silky single strands, lays flat				Receding	
Lanugo	None on face, present on body				Present on shoulders				No lanugo	
Labia & Clitoris	Prominent clitoris, labia small, widely separated		Labia majora larger, nearly cover clitoris				Labia minora and clitoris covered			
Testes	Palpable in inguinal canal		In upper scrotum				In lower scrotum			
Scrotum	Few rugae		Rugae anterior portion				Rugae cover		Pendulous	
Skull firmness	Soft to 1" from ant fontanelle	Spongy at edges of fontanelle, center firm			Bones hard, sutures easily displaced				Hard, can't displace	

Examiner's Signature

Placenta Examination Form

Name of Mother_____ EDD: _____

Name of Infant _____

Date of birth _____ Time of birth: _____

Significant health history _____
_____

Brief summary of the birth _____

Length of 3rd stage_____

Method of placental birth:

          Spontaneous _____ Assisted _____ Extracted _____

If extracted, state reasons, method and outcome
_____
_____

Were oxytocic's, either herbal or pharmacological used for postpartum bleeding or to release the placenta?

Yes _____ No _____ If yes, what and why
_____
_____

   Dose_____ Frequency _____

   Results: _____

Total blood loss _____

Before birth of placenta _____

After birth of placenta _____

Retroplacental clots _____ Size _____ Number _____ Placement _____

Approximate age of clots _____ Size and weight _____

Notes:
_____
_____
_____

Placenta Weight _____
Circumference _____
Thickness _____
Color _____

Any signs or symptoms of infection _____ Odor _____ Pallor _____ Other
_____

Maternal (Duncan) side:
Color _____
Consistency: Normal _____ Soft _____ Firm _____
If not complete describe: _____
Overall impression: Infarcts, calcification, abnormalities of the vascular bed, nodes
etc.

_____
_____
_____

Baby's side (Shultz): Overall impression

_____
_____
_____

 Note obvious variations or abnormalities of shape

_____
_____

Extraplacental membranes:
Are the membranes complete: Yes ___ No ___
Presence of Amnion _____
Presence of Chorion _____
Evidence of amniotic web syndrome _____
Point of rupture: Evidence of low lying placental implantation: Yes _____ No _____
Circummarginate _____
Circumvallate _____

Umbilical cord: Site of insertion:

Central ____

Eccentric ____

Battledore _____

        If it is a battledore insertion, where is the point of rupture _____

Velamentous _____

Furcate insertion _____

Evidence of Vasa Previa _____

Cord length _____

True knot(s) _____

False knot(s) _____

Webbing _____

Presence of Warton's jelly _____

Thrombosis _____

Single artery _____ If yes, which artery is missing: right _____ left _____

Chirality of cord: right spiral ___ left spiral ___ none ____ excessive _____

Edema of the cord: Yes ___ No ___

Nuchal cord _____

Sketch a diagram of anything of note:

Overall health and well-being of this newborn

_____
_____
_____
_____

Any evidence of problems with this newborn related to anomalies within this placenta: Yes ___ No ___
If yes explain:

_____
_____
_____
_____

Photographs taken for documentation _____

Referral or consultation: Yes _____ No _____
If yes, with whom _____

_____   _____
Signature of attending midwife   Date

_____   _____
Signature of Consultant – if consult done   Date

Please note: Obvious abnormalities of the placenta may warrant further examination by a pathologist. If you feel that there may be a need for this, do not freeze the placenta. Dry it well, place it in a zip lock bag removing all of the air possible and then place it into an air tight plastic container. Tape it closed with red tape. This is a safe way to transport "Hazardous Biological Waste" if you need to take it for examination to a hospital. Freezing the placenta changes the tissues altering the pathologist's ability to do accurate microscopic examinations.

Client's Name_____ Date Birth_____

	36-48 hours	5 days	2 weeks	4-6 weeks
Time/ Date			.	
T | P | BP				
Feedings milk in nipples sore engorged redness	Breast _____ Formula_____	Breast _____ Formula_____	Breast _____ Formula_____	Breast _____ Formula_____
Involution after pains				
Locia abn odor	#_____ of kotex day Rubra Serosa Alba	#_____ of kotex day Rubra Serosa Alba	#_____ of kotex day Rubra Serosa Alba	#_____ of kotex day Rubra Serosa Alba
Perineum				
Elimination void / BM hemorrhoids discomfort				
Hygiene				
Condition		Hemo_____	Hemo_____	
Midwife				

Baby's Name_____ Wt at birth ___lbs ___oz ____grams

General Condition				
Weight				
Color/Skin				
Umbilicus				
Voiding/BM				
Midwife				
PKU	Date done_____ Days postpartum_____ With whom_____ Results_____			

Postpartum Follow Up Sheet for _____

Baby's Name_____ Date of Birth_____

Date	Issues Discussed	Midwife	Student

Postpartum Follow Up Sheet for _____

Baby's Name_____ Date of Birth_____

Date	Issues Discussed	Midwife	Student

Postpartum Follow Up Sheet for _____

Baby's Name_____ Date of Birth_____

Date	Issues Discussed	Midwife	Student

STATEMENT OF BIRTH

Date of Birth: _____/_____/_____ Time of Birth: _____

Address of Birth: _____

Child's Name: _____ Gender: _____

Mother's Name: _____ Age: _____

Attendant's Name and Title: _____

WITNESSES OTHER THAN ATTENDANT: (If any)

1) Name:_____

    Address: _____

    Relationship to Mother: _____

2) Name:_____

    Address: _____

    Relationship to Mother: _____

I, _____ do hereby swear that all information given in this document is true and accurate to the best of my knowledge.

Date: _____

Attendant Signature: _____

Mother Signature: _____

Witness 1 – Signature: _____

Witness 2 – Signature: _____

Attendant Contact Info:

Name: _____ Phone: _____ Fax: _____

Address:

Summary of Labor, Birth, Immediate Postpartum & Newborn

Client _____

___P___SAB___TAB___L___ VBAC ___ EDD_____ Wks_____ GBS_____ Total Weight Gain:_____

First Stage Summary

Onset latent labor ____/____/____ _____am/pm _____hrs _____min

Onset active labor ____/____/____ _____am/pm _____hrs _____min

Comments:

ROM at ____/____/____ _____am/pm
until delivery _____hrs _____min
Confirmed by □ visual □ nitrazine □ fetal hair □ fern □ referral
Labor Aids
□ ambulant □ positional □ nipple stim □ water □ castor oil
□ enema □ homeopathics □ herbs □ other _____
Membranes □ SROM □ AROM why?_____
With– □ no ctx □ latent □ active □ 2nd stage □ in caul
Amount-- □ fetal hair □ fern □ referral
Condition–□ clear □ lt mec □ mod mec □ thick mec □ term mec

Second Stage Summary

Onset 2nd stage ____/____/____ _____am/pm _____hrs _____min

Birth of Baby ____/____/____ Time of Birth _____am/pm

Resuscitation/Suctioning □ None □ YES
DeLee □ Bulb Syringe □ PPV _____ # of minutes

Comments:

Positions √ Pushed ■ Delivered
□ squat □ stand □ H&K □ McRoberts □ knee/chest
□ lithotomy □ Simms □ on toilet □ waterbirth □ other_____
Presentation □ OA □ OP □ Other _____
Nuchal Arm □ none x_____ **Nuchal Cord** □ none x_____

Perineum □ TEAR □ EPIS □ intact □ <1 □ 1 □ 2 □ 3 □ 4
Labial Tear □ intact □ skids □ needed sutures
Repair □ YES □ NO
by_____

Third Stage Summary

Placenta Delivered ____/____/____ _____am/pm _____hrs _____min
Was Delivered □ spontaneously □ assisted □ manual removal
Placenta Birthed in □ Shultz □ Duncan
Placenta/Membranes □ complete □ incom □ unsure □ cord 3 vessel
cord □ stained □ marginal □ velamentous □ TRUE/FALSE knots
calcifications □ small □ average □ large
Comments:

Herbs_____
@_____am/pm @_____am/pm

Estimated PBL _____cups/cc □ scant □ moderate □ heavy
(0-250cc/1c) (250-1000 cc/1-4 c) (>1000cc/4c)

Newborn Examination   ♀   ♂

Date of Examination_____ Time _____am/pm

Baby's Name _____

Weight _____lbs _____oz _____gm
Length_____ Chest_____ OFC_____
EGA by dates_____ EGA by exam_____wks

Eye Care (Erythromycin) □ refused □ administered time_____am/pm
Vit K □ refused □ advised □ admin □ IM □ PO BY_____
Cord Blood □ blood type/rh □ RPR □ HIV □ Hep B □ other _____

Comments_____
Examination by_____ Apgars 1min_____5min_____

Reflexes □ moro □ plantar □ palmar □ Babinski □ suck
□ root/suck □ blink □ stepping

Physical Exam √ if WNL

□ gen appearance _____	□ nipples_____
□ skin/color_____	□ abdomen_____
□ fontanels_____	□ cord_____
□ head_____	□ spine_____
□ ears_____	□ anus_____
□ eyes_____	□ genitalia_____
□ nose_____	□ extremities_____
□ throat_____	□ hips_____
□ mouth_____	□ birth marks_____
□ clavicle_____	□ mongolian spot_____
□ heart_____	□ stork bite_____
□ lungs_____	

Client Discharged / Midwife Left

Date_____ Time _____am/pm _____hrs _____min pp

Total PPBL _____cups/cc Midwife_____
Comments:

Present @ Birth

Midwife_____

Asst_____

Others_____

Transport Summary

Client

Name_____ Age_____ G___ P___ A___ L___ Phone (____)_____
Address_____ City _____ State_____ Zip_____
Emergency Contact _____ Phone (____)_____ Relation_____
LMP_____EDD_____ Dates changed_____ by_____
Prenatal care began _____ @ _____wks Number of visits with MW____ other____
Blood type_____ HBG_____ Antibody screen_____ RPR/VDRL_____ Rubella_____ Pap_____
GBS_____ GC/CT_____ HIV_____ Heb B_____ Glucose_____

Labor

Latent labor began Date_____ Time_____ am/pm FHR _____
Active labor began Date_____ Time_____ am/pm FHR _____
Rupture of membranes Date_____ Time_____ am/pm Color _____ INTACT
Assessment prior to transport: Temp_____ Pulse_____ Resps_____ B/P_____ Laceration_____
_____cm _____eff _____station Position of baby_____ Urine Prot____ Gluc____ Ket____ Nit____
Placenta time_____ am/pm Complete YES NO   EBL _____cups/cc
Reason for transport_____
_____

Newborn

Date of Birth_____ Time_____am/pm
Weight _____lbs _____oz _____grams
Meconium_____ Eye care_____ Vit K_____
Bulb_____Delee_____ Bag & mask_____ CPR_____
Reason for transport_____
_____
_____

Apgars of Baby			
	1 min	5 min	10 min
Heart	0 1 2	0 1 2	0 1 2
Resps	0 1 2	0 1 2	0 1 2
Reflex	0 1 2	0 1 2	0 1 2
Tone	0 1 2	0 1 2	0 1 2
Color	0 1 2	0 1 2	0 1 2

Transport

_____Hospital contacted on_____ at _____am/pm DR_____
by EMS – Date called _____ at _____ am/pm Arrived @_____ departed @_____
by Private vehicle- departed on _____ at _____ am/pm Arrived @_____

Midwife's Name:_____ Signature_____